Martial Arts Adventures:

Tales of Courage and Mastery

Written By

Donald P Mathews

ISBN: 978-1-312-44515-4

Printed by Lulu.com

Cover design by Donald P Mathews

Printed in the U.S.A.

Dedication

To Janet, Thank you for your unwavering support, encouragement, and belief in the power of dreams. Your presence in my life has been a constant source of inspiration, and I am grateful for your love and guidance. This book is dedicated to you, a true champion of bravery and resilience.

And to Grace, My faithful companion and source of unconditional love. Your joyful spirit and unwavering loyalty have brought much joy into my life. Thank you for always being by my side, offering comfort and companionship during the creative journey.

Together, Janet and Grace, you have played an integral role in shaping the stories within these pages. May this book serve as a testament to our shared belief in the strength of the human spirit and the power of embracing one's unique path.

With all my love and appreciation,

Don

Introduction

Embark on an exhilarating journey through the pages of this action-packed collection of stories, "Martial Arts Adventures: Tales of Courage and Mastery." Join four courageous and unlikely heroes as they discover their hidden potential, face thrilling challenges, and prove that true strength comes from within.

In "The Martial Arts Mouse: A Tale of Bravery," join Milo, a curious and brave mouse, as he embarks on a heroic quest to become a skilled warrior. Experience the captivating story of Milo's unwavering bravery, relentless pursuit of martial arts mastery, and the ultimate battle against a formidable foe to protect his village.

Prepare for "The Kickboxing Kangaroo's Challenge," a thrilling adventure featuring Kaden, a spirited kangaroo with a passion for kickboxing. Follow Kaden's journey as he confronts his fears, trains tirelessly, and faces a daunting challenge that will test his skills and determination like never before.

Uncover "The Little Ninja's Secret" as young Hiro embraces his destiny as a ninja, despite his small stature. Delve into the secrets of the ancient ninja arts as Hiro navigates treacherous obstacles, uncovers hidden truths, and battles against the forces of darkness to protect his village.

In "The Samurai Squirrel's Samurai Skills," witness the inspiring tale of Hiroshi, a determined squirrel with a deep admiration for the noble samurai warriors. Follow Hiroshi's path as he trains under the wise Sensei Takeshi, mastering the art of the samurai and defending his forest home from danger.

Each of these captivating stories weaves together elements of courage, discipline, and the power of self-belief. Through their trials and triumphs, these unlikely heroes teach us the importance of perseverance, teamwork, and embracing our unique strengths.

Whether you are a fan of samurai tales, ninja adventures, kickboxing showdowns, or tales of bravery, "Martial Arts Adventures: Tales of Courage and Mastery." promises to transport readers of all ages into a world filled with excitement, inspiration, and the enduring spirit of martial arts. Get ready to be enthralled by these unforgettable tales that remind us that anyone, regardless of size or species, can achieve greatness through determination, courage, and mastery of their chosen path.

Table of Contents

Page 10

"The Martial Arts Mouse: A Tale of Bravery"

Page 21

"The Kickboxing Kangaroo's Challenge"

Page 32

"The Little Ninja's Secret"

Page 41

"The Samurai Squirrel's Samurai Skills"

The Martial Arts Mouse:

A Tale of Bravery

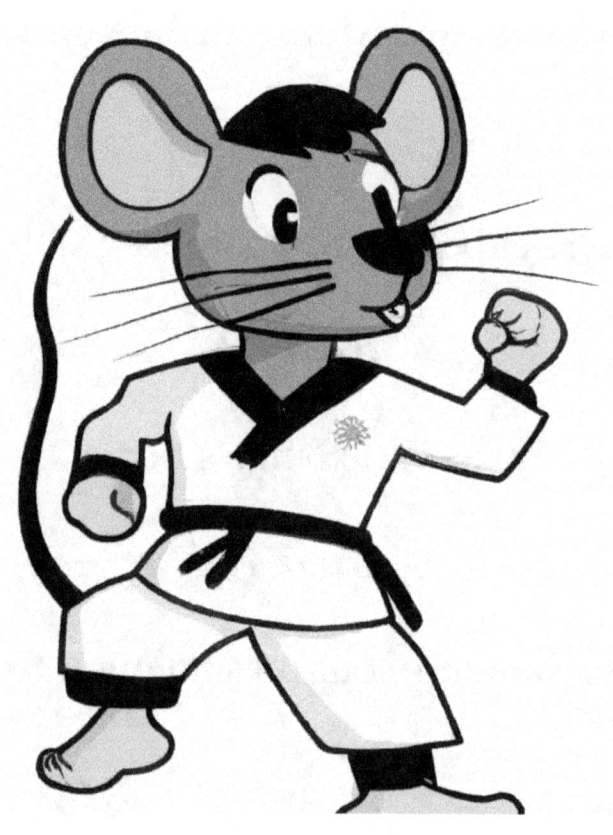

In a quaint little mouse village nestled beneath a towering oak tree, there lived a curious and brave little mouse named Milo. With his bright eyes and a heart full of determination, Milo had always dreamt of becoming a great warrior. While his fellow mice scurried about their daily chores, Milo would often be found practicing his moves and imagining grand adventures.

One sunny morning, as Milo ventured into the village library, he stumbled upon a dusty old book hidden on the highest shelf. The book had a soft cover with golden letters that read, "The Legends of Martial Arts Masters." Milo's whiskers twitched with excitement as he carefully opened the book, revealing an ancient scroll hidden within its pages.

The scroll depicted a legendary mouse warrior, garbed in a flowing robe and wielding a staff with incredible prowess. Milo's heart raced with anticipation as he read the scroll's inscription:

"To unlock the path of bravery and become a true warrior, seek the wisdom of Master Shen in the faraway Bamboo Forest."

Milo's mind filled with determination, and he knew that this was his chance to embark on a remarkable journey. With the scroll tucked safely into his satchel, he hurried back home to prepare for the adventure ahead.

As Milo gathered some provisions for his journey, his best friend, Oliver, scurried over with a mischievous glint in his eye. Oliver was an older and wiser mouse known for his quick wit and clever advice.

"Milo, my friend, where are you off to with such excitement?" Oliver inquired, raising an eyebrow curiously.

Milo beamed, unable to contain his enthusiasm. "Oliver, I've discovered an ancient scroll that reveals the path to bravery and becoming a warrior! I will find Master Shen in the Bamboo Forest and train to become a martial arts mouse!"

Oliver chuckled, patting Milo on the back. "Ah, Milo, your dreams know no bounds. But remember, bravery is not just about fighting skills. It is about courage, resilience, and the willingness to face your fears. May your journey be filled with wisdom and strength."

Milo nodded, appreciating Oliver's wisdom. He bid farewell to his family and friends with his satchel filled with provisions, setting off on his grand adventure.

Days turned into weeks as Milo traveled through lush meadows, crossed babbling brooks, and trekked through dense forests. Finally, on the horizon, he caught sight of the magnificent Bamboo Forest, its tall stalks swaying gently in the breeze.

Milo noticed a mysterious figure observing him from the shadows as he entered the forest. It was a wise and elderly owl named Ophelia, known as the guardian of the Bamboo Forest.

"Welcome, young mouse. I have been awaiting your arrival," Ophelia hooted, her eyes filled with ancient wisdom. "To find Master Shen, you must pass the trials of the Bamboo Forest. Only those with bravery and determination can unlock its secrets."

Milo's heart fluttered with a mix of excitement and nervousness. He steeled himself, ready to face whatever challenges awaited him.

Milo ventured deeper into the Bamboo Forest, the air thick with anticipation. He encountered a series of trials designed to test his resolve and courage.

The first trial was a daunting obstacle course, where Milo had to navigate through winding paths, leap over fallen logs, and balance on narrow branches. With each challenge, his confidence grew, and he pushed himself to go beyond his limits.

In the second trial, Milo faced a wise old turtle named Master Koji, renowned for his formidable martial arts skills. Master Koji presented Milo with a wooden staff and challenged him to defend himself against a series of swift attacks. Though Milo was smaller and less experienced, his agility and quick reflexes surprised Master Koji and himself.

The final trial awaited Milo at the heart of the Bamboo Forest. A massive waterfall cascaded into a serene pool, its waters shimmering with hidden power. Milo knew that he had to dive into the pool and retrieve a sacred stone hidden at the bottom to prove his bravery.

Summoning his courage, Milo took a deep breath and plunged into the icy waters. He swam against the current, his tiny paws propelling him forward with unwavering determination. Just as his strength waned, he saw the sacred stone. He grasped it tightly with one final surge of energy and resurfaced triumphantly.

Emerging from the pool, Milo stood before a grand oak tree with ancient engravings. The ground rumbled as he touched the sacred stone to the tree's bark, and the mighty branches parted, revealing a hidden chamber.

Inside the chamber, Milo found himself face to face with Master Shen, an elderly mouse with a gentle smile and eyes sparkling with wisdom.

"Welcome, young warrior. Your journey and trials have led you here," Master Shen greeted Milo warmly. "To become a true martial arts mouse, you must not only hone your physical skills but also nurture your inner strength and embrace compassion."

Milo listened intently as Master Shen shared stories of courage, discipline, and the power of kindness. Under Master Shen's tutelage, Milo trained diligently, refining his techniques and channeling his bravery into a force for good.

Months passed, and Milo's skills flourished under the guidance of Master Shen. He learned the art of balance, the precision of strikes, and the importance of inner peace. But above all, he discovered the true meaning of bravery—courage that stemmed from a place deep within his heart.

One fateful day, word reached the Bamboo Forest of a distressed village. It was Milo's village, under threat from a menacing group of rats led by a tyrannical rat king. Without hesitation, Milo knew it was time to test his newfound bravery and face the ultimate challenge.

Milo returned to his village, accompanied by Master Shen and the wisdom of the Bamboo Forest. Initially startled by Milo's transformation, the villagers soon saw the bravery radiating from their once-timid friend.

The battle raged as Milo and his fellow mice fought valiantly against the rat invaders. Milo's lightning-fast strikes and agile maneuvers inspired the villagers, filling them with renewed hope.

With Master Shen's guidance, Milo confronted the rat king in a showdown that echoed through the village. Milo's bravery and unwavering determination prevailed as the sun set on the battlefield. The rat king was defeated, and peace was restored to the town.

In the aftermath of the battle, the villagers gathered to honor Milo and celebrate his bravery. Milo stood before them, humbled by their admiration but knowing that true bravery was not a solitary act. It was a collective effort born from the courage and unity of all who fought alongside him.

Oliver, his loyal friend, approached him with a gleam in his eye. "Milo, my dear friend, you have embodied bravery. Your journey has taught us all that courage lies within, waiting to be unleashed."

Milo smiled, grateful for the lessons he had learned and the friends he had made along the way. From that day forward, he dedicated himself to sharing martial arts wisdom and inspiring others to discover their courage.

And so, the legend of Milo, the Martial Arts Mouse, spread far and wide, reminding everyone that bravery knows no boundaries. The extraordinary can arise in the hearts of the small and the humble.

Remember, dear reader, within you lies bravery waiting to be awakened. Like Milo, embrace your fears, nurture your strength, and embark on your journey of self-discovery and courage.

The Kickboxing

Kangaroo's Challenge

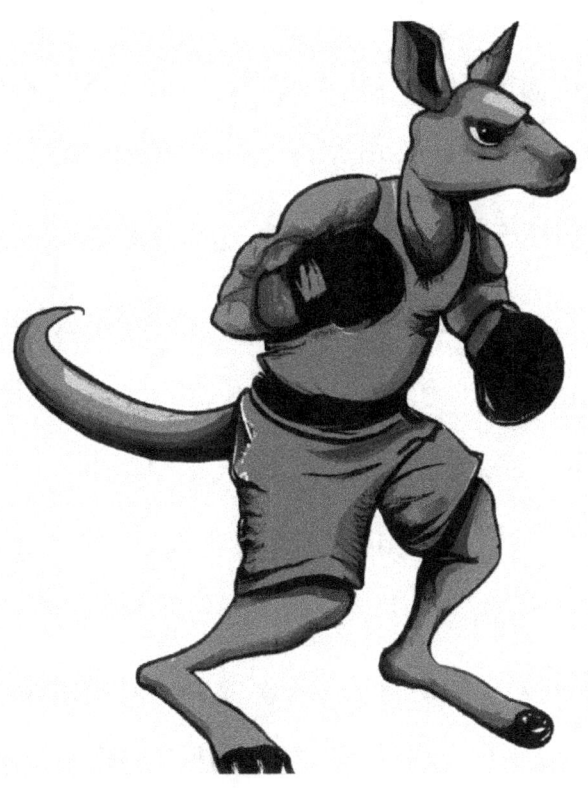

In the vast expanse of the Australian outback, amidst the red desert and towering eucalyptus trees, lived a kickboxing kangaroo named Kaden. Known for his impressive speed and agility, Kaden had mastered the art of kickboxing like no other kangaroo in the land. He spent his day's training and honing his skills, always seeking new challenges to test his limits.

One fine morning, as the sun painted the sky with hues of orange and gold, Kaden stumbled upon an old, weathered parchment hidden beneath a eucalyptus tree. As he unrolled it, a message written in elegant calligraphy caught his eye: "The Ultimate Kickboxing Challenge awaits those who seek glory and triumph. Follow the path to the mystical Dojo of Champions to prove your skills."

Excitement surged through Kaden's veins. He knew this was his chance to take his kickboxing prowess to the next level. With the parchment safely tucked in his pouch, he bounded off, determined to embark on an extraordinary journey.

As Kaden traversed the sprawling landscape, his powerful legs carrying him effortlessly, he came across a wise old wombat named Wilbur. Wilbur was renowned for his wisdom and was known to guide wanderers in the outback.

Curiosity sparked in Wilbur's eyes as he noticed the determined expression on Kaden's face. "Ah, young kickboxing kangaroo, I sense a fire burning within you. What brings you on this path of adventure?" Wilbur inquired; his voice filled with a hint of excitement.

Kaden grinned, unable to contain his enthusiasm. "Wise Wombat, I have discovered a parchment that leads me to the Dojo of Champions. I seek to prove myself and take on the Ultimate Kickboxing Challenge."

Wilbur nodded sagely, his whiskers twitching. "Ah, the Dojo of Champions is a place of immense skill and competition. To reach it, you must undertake a perilous journey. But be warned, young one, the road to glory is often fraught with challenges that test your physical strength and spirit."

With newfound determination, Kaden bid farewell to Wilbur and continued his journey, his heart resolute and his muscles primed for the trials that awaited him.

As Kaden ventured further into the outback, the scorching sun beat down upon him, intensifying the dry heat of the desert. Determined, he pressed on, determined to prove himself worthy of the Ultimate Kickboxing Challenge.

Suddenly, a swirling sandstorm erupted, obscuring his vision and sending him stumbling. Kaden fought against the elements, his powerful kicks and swift movements slicing through the gusts of wind. With every step, he grew stronger, his resolve unyielding.

Emerging from the sandstorm, Kaden found himself face to face with a group of desert-dwelling kangaroos. They were skilled fighters known for their lightning-fast strikes and evasive maneuvers. Clearly, they were the gatekeepers of the desert, guarding the path to the Dojo of Champions.

One of the kangaroos, a fierce and battle-hardened warrior named Karina, stepped forward. "To prove your worth, you must defeat each of us in combat," she declared, her voice tinged with challenge.

Kaden nodded, prepared to face the trials that lay before him. He unleashed his formidable kickboxing skills with each opponent, evading strikes and countering with precision and finesse. The battles were intense, but Kaden's determination and perseverance carried him through.

After a series of hard-fought victories, Karina, impressed by Kaden's skills and unwavering spirit, bowed respectfully. "You have shown great skill and resilience, young kangaroo. You may continue your journey to the Dojo of Champions. May you find the glory you seek."

As Kaden ventured further into the outback, he entered a dense forest, where ancient gum trees whispered secrets of battles fought, and legends forged. The majestic Dojo of Champions stood in the heart of the forest, a place of training and enlightenment for warriors from all corners of the world.

As Kaden entered the grand gates of the Dojo, he was greeted by the Chief Instructor, Master Hiroshi, a wise and revered kangaroo who had dedicated his life to the art of kickboxing.

"Welcome, young warrior," Master Hiroshi said, his voice resonating with authority. "To prove yourself worthy of the Ultimate Kickboxing Challenge, you must train under my guidance and face opponents who will push your limits. Only then can you claim victory."

Eager to learn and grow, Kaden immersed himself in the rigorous training regimen of the Dojo. Under Master Hiroshi's watchful eye, he perfected his technique, refining his kicks, punches, and footwork. Days turned into weeks and weeks into months as Kaden absorbed the wisdom and teachings of the Dojo.

Months of training passed, and Kaden's skills reached new heights. The time had come for him to face the ultimate test—the Final Showdown.

In the Dojo's grand arena, Kaden stood opposite his opponent, a formidable and renowned kickboxing kangaroo named Ryu. The air crackled with anticipation as the crowd gathered, eager to witness the clash of titans.

Ryu, his muscles rippling with power, eyed Kaden with a mixture of respect and intensity. "You have come far, young one. Show me what you have gotten," he challenged, his voice filled with the echoes of countless battles.

With adrenaline coursing through his veins, Kaden focused his mind and centered his spirit. The battle that ensued was a symphony of skill, agility, and sheer willpower. Each kick and punch carried the weight of their journey, dreams, and unwavering determination.

The crowd erupted in thunderous applause as Kaden's swift moves and relentless determination led him to victory. At that moment, he realized that the true challenge was not just about winning but about discovering his strength.

As Kaden basked in the glory of his triumph, he realized that the Ultimate Kickboxing Challenge was not merely a physical competition. It was a journey of self-discovery, resilience, and the pursuit of excellence.

With newfound wisdom, Kaden returned to his home in the outback; his heart filled with gratitude for the challenges that had shaped him. He became a mentor to aspiring kickboxing kangaroos, sharing his knowledge and inspiring them to embrace their unique strengths.

Years passed, and Kaden's name became legendary throughout the land. His legacy as the kickboxing kangaroo who had overcome countless trials lived on, inspiring generations to never back down from a challenge and to always fight for their dreams.

And so, dear reader, remember the tale of Kaden, the kickboxing kangaroo, and let it remind us that the most significant challenges are often the catalysts for our greatest victories. Embrace the challenges that come your way, for within them lies the potential for greatness.

The Little Ninja's Secret

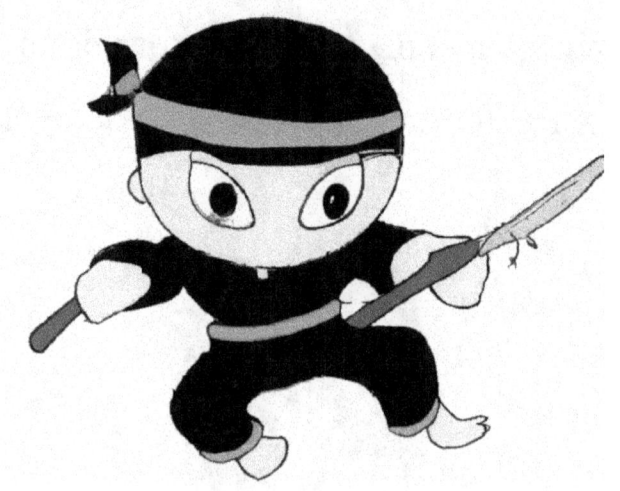

A young boy named Hiro lived in a small village nestled amidst rolling hills and cherry blossom trees. While Hiro appeared to be an ordinary child, he held a secret known only to a select few—he was a little ninja.

By day, Hiro attended school and played with his friends, blending seamlessly into the crowd. But when night fell, and the moon shone brightly, Hiro would slip away into the shadows, training rigorously in the ancient art of ninjutsu.

Hidden within his humble home was a secret training room adorned with traditional weaponry and adorned with scrolls containing the wisdom of generations. It was here that Hiro honed his skills, guided by the teachings of his ancestors.

Hiro's training had always been a solitary pursuit until one fateful day when he stumbled upon an old scroll that revealed the existence of a legendary ninja master known as Sensei Takeshi.

Sensei Takeshi was said to possess incredible knowledge and skill, and it was believed that he could awaken the true potential of any aspiring ninja.

Filled with curiosity and a burning desire to learn, Hiro embarked on a journey to seek out Sensei Takeshi. Through treacherous terrain and across raging rivers, Hiro braved the perils of the unknown until he finally arrived at a hidden mountain retreat.

There, he met Sensei Takeshi, a wise and seasoned master, who agreed to take Hiro under his wing. Under Sensei Takeshi's guidance, Hiro's training took on a new level of intensity and purpose. Sensei Takeshi taught Hiro the physical aspects of ninjutsu and instilled in him the importance of discipline, respect, and compassion.

As Hiro delved deeper into his training, Sensei Takeshi introduced him to the concept of secrets. The little ninja learned that secrets were not merely meant to be hidden but were valuable tools to be wielded with wisdom.

Sensei Takeshi explained, "A true ninja understands the power of secrets. They can be used to protect and preserve, to surprise and confound. But remember, Hiro, secrets carry great responsibility. They must be used wisely and never for personal gain."

With this newfound understanding, Hiro learned to embrace the secret nature of his training. He revealed that he possessed ancient techniques and strategies unknown to the world.

Sensei Takeshi believed that true mastery could only be achieved by facing one's greatest fears. To test Hiro's progress, he devised a trial known as the Test of Shadows. It required Hiro to navigate a labyrinthine maze filled with traps and obstacles, all while remaining unseen by the watchful eyes of the temple guards.

As Hiro ventured into the dimly lit maze, he relied on his heightened senses and trained instincts. His breath echoed in his ears as he moved like a whisper, swiftly and silently. With each step, he demonstrated his understanding of stealth and patience.

After what felt like an eternity, Hiro emerged from the labyrinth, completing the Test of Shadows. Sensei Takeshi smiled proudly, acknowledging Hiro's growth and readiness to face more significant challenges.

Hiro's training with Sensei Takeshi continued, pushing him to new heights of skill and mental fortitude. But little did he know that darkness loomed on the horizon.

An ancient ninja clan, long thought to be extinct, emerged from the shadows, seeking to obtain the secret techniques held within Hiro's village. Led by the sinister Master Ryu, they launched a ruthless attack, leaving devastation in their wake.

Sensei Takeshi, recognizing the threat, made the difficult decision to entrust Hiro with a crucial mission—to protect the village and its people from the clutches of the ruthless clan. Hiro knew the time had come for him to use his skills for a greater purpose.

Hiro's heart raced as he confronted Master Ryu, his nemesis, atop a moonlit hill. The clash between light and darkness was about to unfold, and the fate of Hiro's village hung in the balance.

With every strike and evasion, Hiro drew upon his training and the teachings of Sensei Takeshi. He fought for himself and the ideals of honor, justice, and protection.

Hiro's resilience and unwavering spirit shone through as the battle raged on. He pushed beyond his limits, displaying mastery that surprised even Master Ryu. The clash of their skills created an awe-inspiring spectacle, but ultimately, Hiro's unwavering belief in the power of good emerged triumphant.

In the aftermath of the battle, Hiro stood before the village, a symbol of hope and inspiration. The people rejoiced, their spirits lifted by the bravery and skill of the little ninja who had protected them.

Sensei Takeshi approached Hiro, a glimmer of pride in his eyes. "You have proven yourself to be a true master of the ninja arts, Hiro. But remember, the journey never ends. As you continue to grow, share your knowledge, and uphold the virtues of a true ninja."

And so, Hiro embraced his role as a protector and mentor, passing on the ancient art of ninjutsu to future generations. His village flourished under the watchful eye of the little ninja, and he was forever grateful for his courage and dedication.

The tale of Hiro, the little ninja, would be told for generations to come—a testament to the power of hidden strengths, the importance of mentors, and the enduring legacy of those who embrace their true calling.

The Samurai Squirrels

Samurai Skills

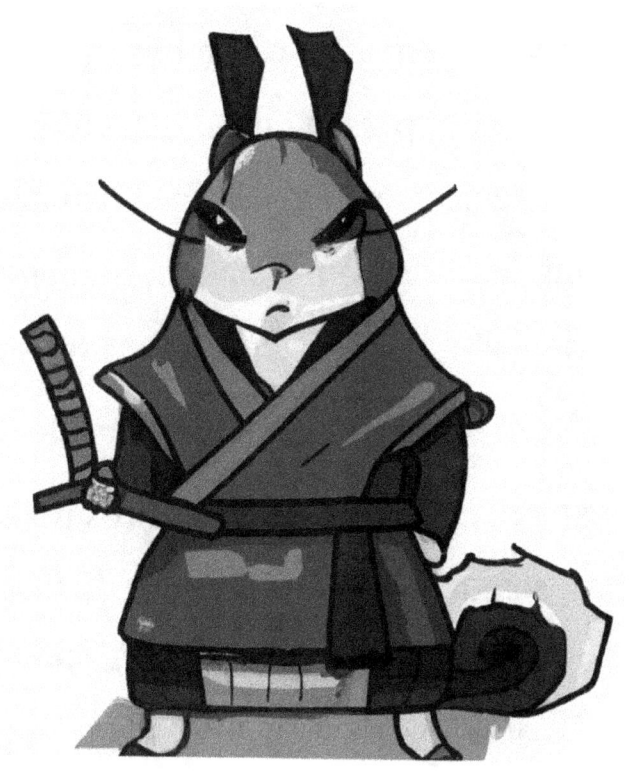

A squirrel named Hiroshi lived in a serene forest nestled between towering trees and babbling brooks. Hiroshi was no ordinary squirrel—he deeply admired the noble samurai warriors and longed to acquire their legendary skills.

Every day, Hiroshi would observe the samurai who occasionally passed through the forest, their elegant movements and disciplined demeanor captivating his attention. He admired their unwavering courage, mastery of the sword, and code of honor.

Inspired by their example, Hiroshi yearned to become a samurai himself. However, he faced a unique challenge—he was a squirrel. But Hiroshi believed that with determination and the guidance of a wise mentor, he could overcome any obstacle.

One day, as Hiroshi scurried through the forest, he encountered an aged tortoise named Sensei Takeshi. Sensei Takeshi was renowned for his wisdom and knowledge of the ancient ways of the samurai.

Hiroshi approached the wise old tortoise and shared his burning desire to become a samurai. Sensei Takeshi listened attentively; his eyes filled with understanding. After reflection, he agreed to become Hiroshi's mentor, guiding him on his quest to acquire samurai skills.

Sensei Takeshi taught Hiroshi the importance of discipline, respect, and inner strength. He explained the Bushido code, the way of the samurai, emphasizing values such as honor, loyalty, and integrity. Hiroshi absorbed these teachings eagerly, eager to embody the virtues of a true samurai.

Under Sensei Takeshi's guidance, Hiroshi embarked on a rigorous training regimen. He learned the art of wielding a samurai sword, honing his balance and precision. Hiroshi also practiced meditation to develop a calm mind and keen focus.

In addition to physical training, Sensei Takeshi taught Hiroshi about the history and philosophy of the samurai. Hiroshi delved into ancient scrolls, studying the tactics and strategies of legendary samurai warriors. He absorbed their wisdom and adapted it to suit his unique squirrel form.

As the days turned weeks and weeks into months, Hiroshi's skills grew, and his determination remained unyielding. He trained tirelessly, practicing his sword techniques, perfecting his balance on narrow tree branches, and sharpening his senses to anticipate his opponents' moves.

Sensei Takeshi believed that true samurai skills were about physical prowess and having an indomitable spirit. To test Hiroshi's courage, he devised a trial that would push the squirrel to his limits.

They ventured deep into the heart of the forest, where a treacherous ravine awaited them. The ravine was infamous for its jagged cliffs and perilous crossing. It required unwavering focus and complete trust in one's abilities.

Hiroshi gazed at the ravine, its depths filled with swirling mist, and felt a mixture of fear and excitement. He took a deep breath, drawing upon his training, and stepped onto the first rock, balancing with delicate precision.

With each step, Hiroshi's confidence grew. The ravine tested his courage, but he remained resolute, channeling the samurai spirit within him. Finally, after what felt like an eternity, Hiroshi reached the other side, victorious.

Sensei Takeshi knew that true samurai skills were tested in combat. He arranged a friendly duel for Hiroshi with a fellow forest dweller—a skilled raccoon named Riku. Riku, too, had trained diligently in the ways of the samurai and was known for his agility and quick reflexes.

As Hiroshi faced Riku in the clearing, the tension between them was palpable. They exchanged formal bows, a sign of mutual respect, and drew their wooden training swords. The duel began, the clashing of their swords echoing through the forest.

Hiroshi's squirrel form allowed him to dart and maneuver with lightning speed, while Riku's raccoon agility allowed him to anticipate Hiroshi's moves. It was a dance of skill, technique, and strategy. They fought with honor and grace, their swords swirling in the air.

The duel reached its climax as Hiroshi, channeling the spirit of the samurai, executed a flawless maneuver, disarming Riku and winning the duel. Despite the intensity of the battle, both Hiroshi and Riku emerged from it with a deeper respect for one another's skills.

Word of Hiroshi's remarkable journey spread throughout the forest, earning him the nickname "The Samurai Squirrel." Animals far and wide marveled at his courage and skill, and many sought his guidance and mentorship.

Hiroshi embraced his role as a teacher, sharing his knowledge and inspiring others to embrace the principles of the samurai. He believed that the path of the samurai was not limited to a specific species—it was a way of life accessible to all who embraced its virtues.

With each passing day, Hiroshi's influence grew, and the forest became a harmonious community that upheld the values of the samurai—honor, respect, and compassion.

Hiroshi's journey as the Samurai Squirrel left a lasting legacy. His teachings were passed down from generation to generation, inspiring countless creatures to embrace the way of the samurai.

The peaceful forest thrived under Hiroshi's guidance, becoming a place of unity and understanding. Animals of all species lived together, respecting one another's differences and embracing the code of honor and integrity.

And so, the tale of the Samurai Squirrel serves as a reminder that true strength lies not in one's physical form but in one's heart and spirit. With determination and guidance, anyone can embody the virtues of the samurai and make a positive impact in the world.

THE

END

www.ingramcontent.com/pod-product-compliance
Lightning Source LLC
Chambersburg PA
CBHW070340290526
45791CB00003B/1403